SMOOTHIES FOR THYROID HEALING

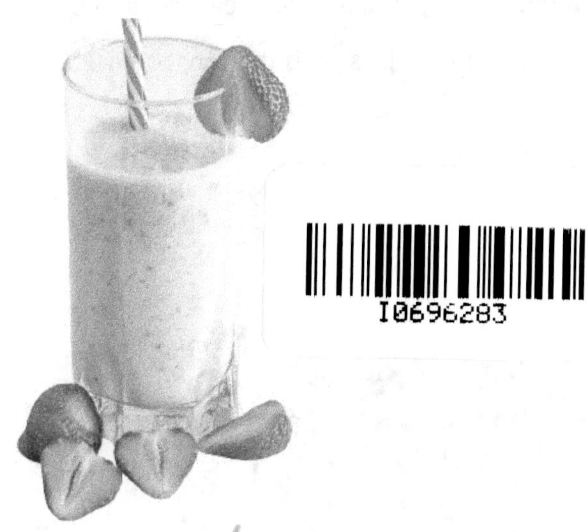

Dr. Kimberly Carlos

Copyright © 2023 by Dr. Kimberly Carlos

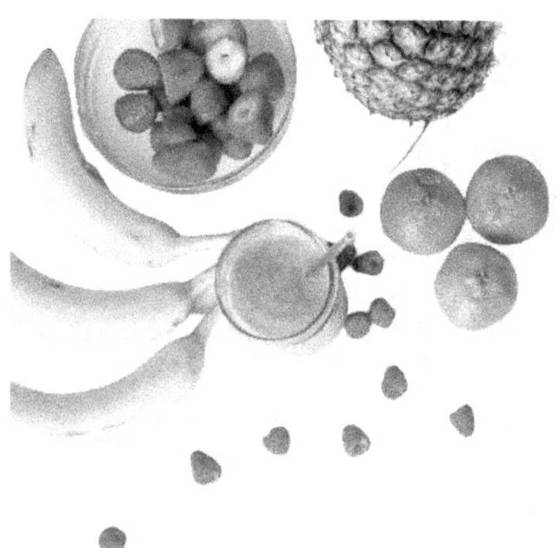

TABLE OF CONTENT

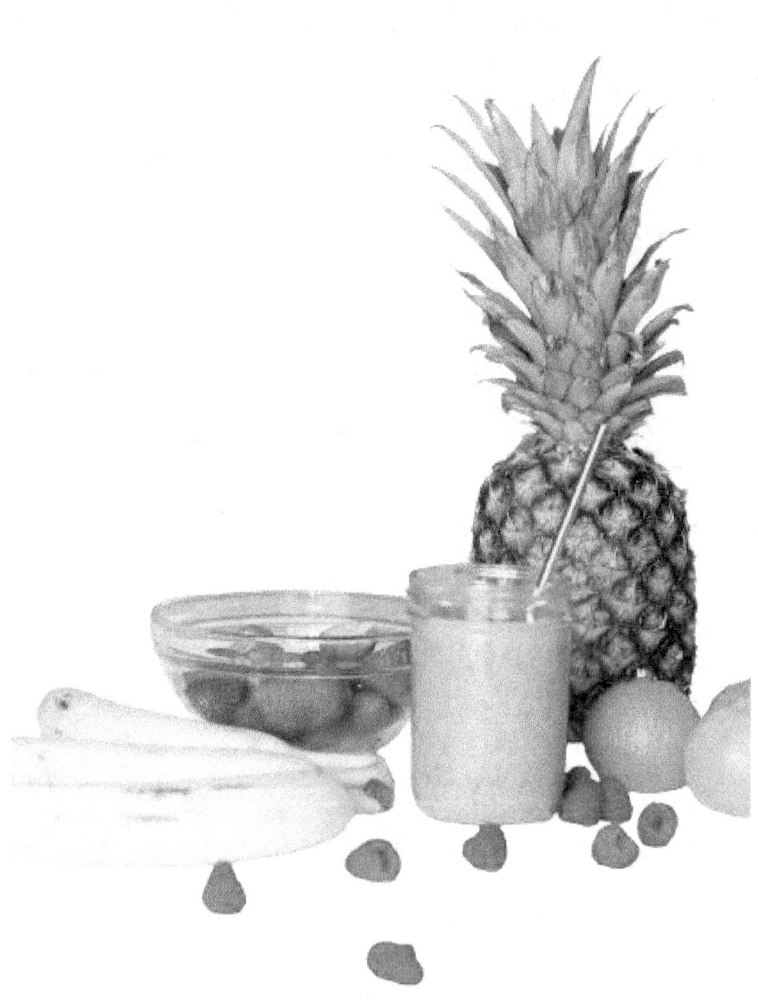

INTRODUCTION

In a quiet village nestled between rolling hills, lived a woman named Maya. She had always been full of life, but a sudden illness cast a shadow over her vibrant spirit. Doctors diagnosed her with thyroid dysfunction, leaving her fatigued and disheartened.

Determined to regain her vitality, Maya embarked on a journey of healing.

One day, as she wandered through the village market, Maya's eyes fell upon a small smoothie stand operated by a friendly woman named Elena.

Intrigued by the vibrant array of fruits, vegetables, and herbs, Maya struck up a conversation. Elena shared stories of her own battles with health issues and how she had harnessed the power of smoothies to heal herself.

Intrigued and hopeful, Maya decided to give it a try. She began incorporating a variety of nutrient-rich ingredients into her daily routine, blending them into delicious concoctions.

Blueberries, rich in antioxidants; spinach, packed with vitamins; and coconut water, known for its hydration properties, became staples in her smoothies.

Weeks turned into months, and Maya's dedication began to pay off. Her energy levels gradually increased, and her enthusiasm for life returned. With each sip of her homemade smoothies, she felt a renewed sense of vitality coursing through her veins. Her thyroid levels started to stabilize, and her doctor was impressed by her progress.

Word spread throughout the village about Maya's journey to health, inspiring others to explore the benefits of smoothies for healing. Elena's little smoothie stand flourished as more villagers sought her guidance and the colorful elixirs she prepared.

Maya's transformation was not just physical; it was a testament to the power of determination, natural remedies, and the support of a caring community. As the village thrived on stories of healing, Maya found herself not only healed but also connected to her neighbors in a profound way.

CHAPTER ONE

Smoothies For Thyroid Healing Diet and Benefits

The thyroid gland plays a crucial role in regulating metabolism, energy production, and overall bodily functions. When the thyroid is out of balance, it can lead to a range of health issues, including fatigue, weight gain, and mood disturbances.

While medical intervention is often necessary, adopting a thyroid-healing diet can provide valuable support to your journey towards optimal health. One effective approach is incorporating nutrient-rich smoothies into your daily routine.

Understanding Thyroid Health and Smoothies' Role

The thyroid gland requires specific nutrients to function optimally. Iodine, selenium, zinc, and certain vitamins are essential for maintaining proper thyroid function. A diet rich in whole foods that provide these nutrients can help support thyroid health.

Smoothies, when carefully crafted with the right ingredients, can deliver a concentrated dose of these essential nutrients.

Blending fruits, vegetables, nuts, seeds, and superfoods can create a powerhouse of nutrients that your body needs to heal and thrive.

Crafting Thyroid-Healing Smoothies: Ingredients and Benefits

1. Iodine-Rich Foods: Incorporating iodine-rich ingredients like sea vegetables (kelp, nori) or using iodized salt is crucial for thyroid health. Iodine is a key component of thyroid hormones, and a deficiency can lead to imbalances. Including a small amount of iodine-rich sea vegetables in your smoothies can provide this essential nutrient.

2. Selenium Sources: Brazil nuts are an excellent source of selenium, a mineral that supports thyroid function and protects the gland from oxidative stress. Adding a couple of Brazil nuts to your smoothie not only imparts a rich, creamy texture but also ensures you receive a dose of this vital nutrient.

3. Leafy Greens: Spinach, kale, and other leafy greens are loaded with vitamins, minerals, and antioxidants. These greens contain iron, which is important for thyroid hormone production and transportation. Including a handful of greens in your smoothie can provide a boost to your thyroid health.

4. Berries and Antioxidants: Blueberries, raspberries, and strawberries are bursting with antioxidants that combat inflammation and oxidative stress. An inflamed thyroid can contribute to thyroid dysfunction, making berries an important addition to your smoothies.

5. Healthy Fats: Avocado, coconut oil, and nuts are sources of healthy fats that support hormone production and absorption of fat-soluble vitamins. These fats can also provide sustained energy and promote satiety.

6. Protein Sources: Adding protein to your smoothies helps maintain steady blood sugar levels and supports muscle repair. Greek yogurt, almond butter, chia seeds, or a scoop of high-quality protein powder can be great choices.

7. Adaptogens: Certain adaptogenic herbs like ashwagandha and holy basil have been linked to improved thyroid function and stress reduction. A small amount of adaptogenic herbs in your smoothie can contribute to overall wellness.

Benefits of a Thyroid-Healing Smoothie Diet

1. Nutrient Boost: Smoothies allow you to easily incorporate a wide variety of nutrient-rich foods into your diet, ensuring your body receives the essential vitamins and minerals it needs for thyroid health.

2. Digestive Ease: Blending ingredients breaks down the cell walls of plants, making their nutrients more accessible and easier to digest, especially for those with thyroid-related digestive issues.

3. Hydration: Many smoothie ingredients, such as fruits and vegetables, have high water content, aiding in hydration—an important factor for overall health and thyroid function.

4. Weight Management: Balanced smoothies can help with weight management by providing a satisfying and nutrient-dense meal or snack option that can curb unhealthy cravings.

5. Convenience: Busy schedules often lead to skipping meals or making unhealthy choices. Smoothies provide a quick, convenient, and wholesome option that supports your thyroid health on the go.

Tips for Creating Effective Thyroid-Healing Smoothies

1. Balance is Key: Aim for a mix of vegetables, fruits, healthy fats, proteins, and superfoods to create a well-rounded smoothie.

2. Mindful Sweeteners: Use natural sweeteners like honey, dates, or maple syrup sparingly to avoid spiking blood sugar levels.

3. Rotate Ingredients: Incorporate a variety of ingredients to ensure you receive a wide range of nutrients and prevent sensitivities.

4. Consult a Professional: If you have a thyroid condition, consult a healthcare professional or registered dietitian before making significant dietary changes.

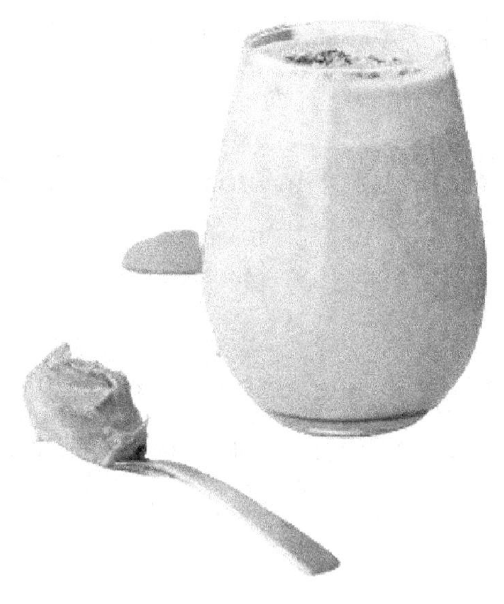

CHAPTER TWO

14-Day Thyroid-Healing Smoothie Plan

Day 1

- Morning Elixir: Start your day with a cleansing green smoothie. Blend spinach, cucumber, celery, a handful of berries, a scoop of plant-based protein powder, and water. Add a sprinkle of chia seeds for added fiber and omega-3 fatty acids.

Day 2

- Tropical Twist: Blend pineapple, mango, coconut water, a small handful of Brazil nuts (for selenium), a splash of lemon juice, and a spoonful of Greek yogurt or a dairy-free alternative.

Day 3

- Berry Blast: Mix blueberries, strawberries, a handful of spinach, almond butter, a tablespoon of ground flaxseeds, and unsweetened almond milk.

Day 4

- Creamy Avocado Delight: Combine avocado, banana, spinach, a scoop of collagen powder, and coconut milk for a creamy and nutrient-rich smoothie.

Day 5

- Iodine Infusion: Blend a mix of greens, cucumber, dulse (a type of seaweed rich in iodine), a handful of berries, and coconut water.

Day 6

- Chia Power: Create a protein-packed smoothie with chia seeds, almond milk, a tablespoon of pumpkin seeds (for zinc), banana, and a pinch of cinnamon.

Day 7

- Citrus Zing: Blend oranges, carrots, a small piece of ginger, a handful of kale, and water for a refreshing and invigorating smoothie.

Day 8

- Nutty Spinach Elixir: Combine spinach, almond milk, a spoonful of almond butter, a date for natural sweetness, and a sprinkle of spirulina (for an extra nutrient boost).

Day 9

- Mixed Berry and Greens Fusion: Mix a variety of berries, a handful of mixed greens (spinach, kale, Swiss chard), flaxseeds, and coconut water.

Day 10

- Golden Turmeric Blend: Blend banana, turmeric (an anti-inflammatory spice), a scoop of vanilla protein powder, a pinch of black pepper (to enhance turmeric absorption), and coconut milk.

Day 11

- Coconut Mango Dream: Combine mango, coconut milk, a small handful of shredded coconut, a scoop of collagen powder, and water.

Day 12

- Antioxidant Boost: Blend acai berries (rich in antioxidants), blueberries, spinach, a tablespoon of hemp seeds (for omega-3s), and almond milk.

Day 13

- Green Energy Booster: Mix kale, cucumber, green apple, a tablespoon of chlorella (a green superfood), lemon juice, and water.

Day 14

- Cocoa-Banana Bliss: Create a satisfying smoothie with banana, raw cacao powder (rich in magnesium), almond butter, a handful of spinach, and your choice of milk.

Tips for Success

1. Stay Hydrated: Alongside your smoothies, drink plenty of water throughout the day to support overall hydration.

2. Variety is Key: Rotate ingredients to ensure you're getting a wide range of nutrients and to prevent palate fatigue.

3. Mindful Ingredients: Choose organic ingredients whenever possible to minimize exposure to pesticides and toxins.

4. Preparation: Prep your ingredients in advance to save time in the morning.

5. Listen to Your Body: Pay attention to how your body responds to different ingredients and adjust as needed.

6. Professional Guidance: If you have a thyroid condition, consult a healthcare professional or registered dietitian before starting any new diet plan.

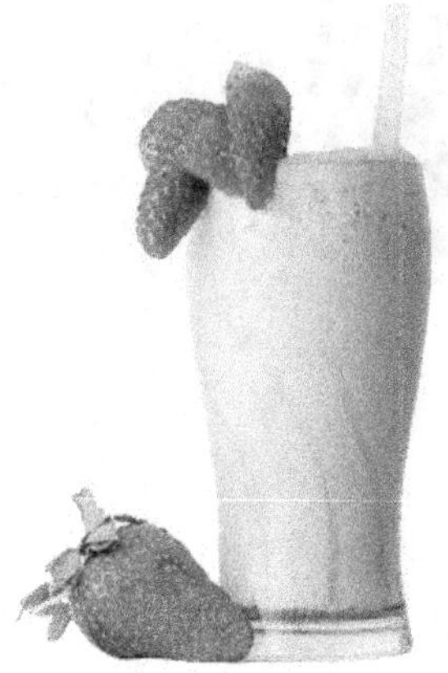

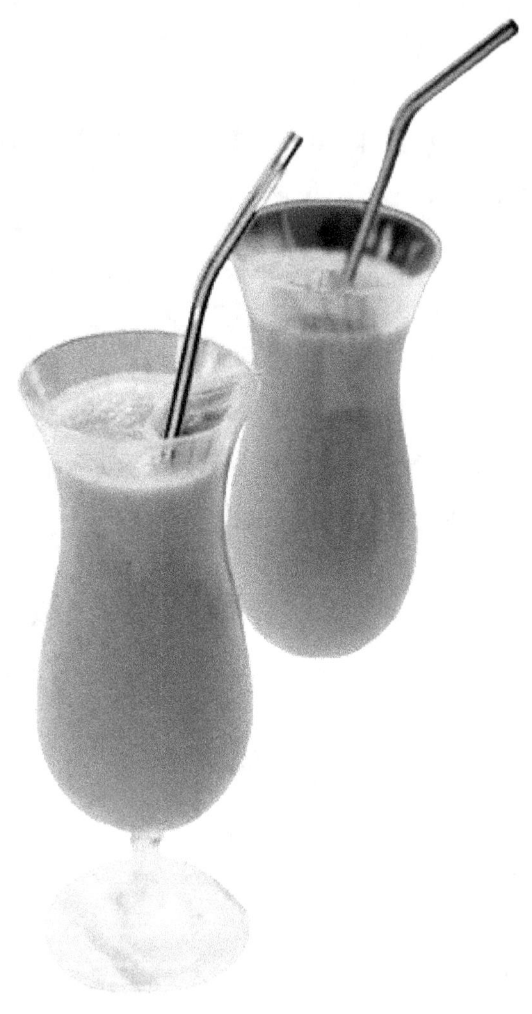

CHAPTER THREE

Thyroid-friendly Smoothie Recipes

1. Vanilla Matcha Elixir

Ingredients:

- 1 teaspoon matcha powder
- 1/2 teaspoon vanilla extract
- 1/2 banana
- 1 cup spinach
- 1 cup almond milk
- 1 teaspoon honey
- Ice cubes

Instructions:

1. Blend matcha powder, vanilla extract, banana, spinach, almond milk, and honey until smooth.

2. Add ice cubes and blend for a refreshing boost.

3. Enjoy the antioxidant-rich goodness of matcha with a touch of vanilla!

Cooking Time: 5 minutes

2. Raspberry Beet Blast

Ingredients:

- 1/2 cup raspberries
- 1/4 cup cooked beets (chopped)
- 1/2 banana
- 1 cup coconut water
- 1 tablespoon flaxseeds
- 1 teaspoon ginger (grated)

Instructions:

1. Blend raspberries, cooked beets, banana, coconut water, flaxseeds, and grated ginger until well mixed.

2. Adjust thickness with more coconut water if desired.

3. Experience the vibrant flavors and colors of raspberries and beets!

Cooking Time: 5 minutes

3. Mango Turmeric Glow

Ingredients:

- 1 cup mango chunks

- 1/2 teaspoon turmeric powder
- 1/2 banana
- 1/2 cup Greek yogurt
- 1/2 cup water
- 1 tablespoon coconut flakes

Instructions:

1. Blend mango chunks, turmeric powder, banana, Greek yogurt, and water until creamy.

2. Sprinkle coconut flakes on top before serving.

3. Embrace the tropical sweetness and anti-inflammatory benefits of turmeric!

Cooking Time: 5 minutes

4. Spirulina Blueberry Boost

Ingredients:

- 1/2 teaspoon spirulina powder
- 1/2 cup blueberries
- 1/2 banana
- 1 cup spinach
- 1 cup coconut water
- 1 tablespoon chia seeds

Instructions:

1. Blend spirulina powder, blueberries, banana, spinach, coconut water, and chia seeds until smooth.

2. Adjust consistency with more coconut water if desired.

3. Energize with the vibrant color and nutrient-rich spirulina!

Cooking Time: 5 minutes

5. Carrot Ginger Vitality

Ingredients:

- 1 carrot (peeled and chopped)
- 1/2 inch ginger (peeled and grated)
- 1/2 banana
- 1/2 cup orange juice
- 1/2 cup water
- 1 tablespoon pumpkin seeds

Instructions:

1. Blend carrot, grated ginger, banana, orange juice, and water until well combined.

2. Add pumpkin seeds and blend briefly.

3. Feel the invigorating power of carrot and ginger!

Cooking Time: 5 minutes

6. Strawberry Basil Refresher

Ingredients:

- 1 cup strawberries
- 1/4 cup fresh basil leaves
- 1/2 banana
- 1/2 cup coconut water
- 1/2 cup almond milk
- Ice cubes

Instructions:

1. Blend strawberries, basil leaves, banana, coconut water, and almond milk until smooth.

2. Add ice cubes and blend for a cool and revitalizing treat.

3. Enjoy the delightful pairing of strawberries and basil!

Cooking Time: 5 minutes

7. Chocolate Cherry Bliss

Ingredients:

- 1/2 cup cherries (pitted)
- 1 tablespoon cocoa powder
- 1/2 banana
- 1 cup almond milk
- 1 tablespoon almonds
- 1 teaspoon honey

Instructions:

1. Blend cherries, cocoa powder, banana, almond milk, almonds, and honey until creamy.

2. Adjust sweetness with more honey if desired.

3. Indulge in the decadent combination of chocolate and cherries!

Cooking Time: 5 minutes

8. Mango Basil Fusion

Ingredients:

- 1 cup mango chunks

- 1/4 cup fresh basil leaves

- 1/2 banana

- 1/2 cup coconut water

- 1/2 cup water

- Ice cubes

Instructions:

1. Blend mango chunks, basil leaves, banana, coconut water, and water until well mixed.

2. Add ice cubes and blend for a refreshing chill.

3. Experience the unique harmony of mango and basil!

Cooking Time: 5 minutes

9. Almond Blueberry Dream

Ingredients:

- 1/2 cup blueberries

- 1/4 cup almonds (soaked overnight)

- 1/2 banana

- 1/2 cup almond milk

- 1 tablespoon honey

- 1/2 teaspoon cinnamon

Instructions:

1. Blend blueberries, soaked almonds, banana, almond milk, honey, and cinnamon until creamy.

2. Adjust sweetness with more honey if desired.

3. Enjoy the nutty essence of almonds with the burst of blueberries!

Cooking Time: 5 minutes

10. Green Mango Spinach

Ingredients:

- 1 cup mango chunks
- 1/2 cup spinach
- 1/2 banana
- 1/2 lime (juiced)
- 1/2 cup coconut water
- Ice cubes

Instructions:

1. Blend mango chunks, spinach, banana, lime juice, coconut water, and ice cubes until smooth.

2. Adjust thickness with more coconut water if desired.

3. Recharge with the tropical zest of mango and the goodness of spinach!

Cooking Time: 5 minutes

11. Golden Pumpkin Spice

Ingredients:

- 1/2 cup cooked pumpkin (chilled)
- 1/2 banana
- 1/2 teaspoon turmeric
- 1/4 teaspoon cinnamon
- 1 cup almond milk
- 1 tablespoon almond butter
- 1 teaspoon honey

Instructions:

1. Blend cooked pumpkin, banana, turmeric, cinnamon, almond milk, almond butter, and honey until creamy.

2. Adjust spices and sweetness to taste.

3. Delight in the warm flavors of pumpkin and spices!

Cooking Time: 5 minutes

12. Raspberry Lemonade Revive

Ingredients:

- 1/2 cup raspberries
- 1 lemon (juiced)
- 1/2 banana
- 1/2 cup coconut water
- 1/2 cup water
- 1 tablespoon fresh mint leaves

Instructions:

1. Blend raspberries, lemon juice, banana, coconut water, and water until smooth.

2. Add fresh mint leaves and blend briefly.

3. Refresh yourself with this zesty and revitalizing blend!

Cooking Time: 5 minutes

13. Spinach Mango Sunshine

Ingredients:

- 1 cup mango chunks
- 1/2 banana
- 1 cup spinach
- 1/2 orange (juiced)
- 1/2 cup water
- Ice cubes

Instructions:

1. Blend mango chunks, banana, spinach, orange juice, and water until well combined.

2. Add ice cubes and blend for a cool, refreshing experience.

3. Bask in the vibrant flavors and colors of this sunshine smoothie!

Cooking Time: 5 minutes

14. Chia Berry Blast

Ingredients:

- 1/2 cup mixed berries (strawberries, blueberries, raspberries)
- 1 tablespoon chia seeds
- 1/2 banana
- 1 cup almond milk
- 1 tablespoon almond butter
- 1 teaspoon honey

Instructions:

1. Blend mixed berries, chia seeds, banana, almond milk, almond butter, and honey until smooth.

2. Adjust sweetness with more honey if desired.

3. Enjoy the burst of berry goodness with added chia power!

Cooking Time: 5 minutes

15. Mango Avocado Euphoria

Ingredients:

- 1 cup mango chunks
- 1/2 avocado
- 1/2 banana
- 1/2 cup coconut water
- 1/2 cup water
- Ice cubes

Instructions:

1. Blend mango chunks, avocado, banana, coconut water, and water until creamy.

2. Add ice cubes and blend for a chilled delight.

3. Experience the creamy indulgence of mango and avocado!

Cooking Time: 5 minutes

16. Pineapple Mint Revitalizer

Ingredients:

- 1/2 cup pineapple chunks
- 1/4 cup fresh mint leaves
- 1/2 banana
- 1/2 lime (juiced)
- 1 cup coconut water
- Ice cubes

Instructions:

1. Blend pineapple chunks, mint leaves, banana, lime juice, coconut water, and ice cubes until smooth.

2. Adjust sweetness with a touch of honey if desired.

3. Feel rejuvenated with the tropical zest of pineapple and mint!

Cooking Time: 5 minutes

17. Cherry Almond Delight

Ingredients:

- 1/2 cup cherries (pitted)
- 1/4 cup almonds (soaked overnight)
- 1/2 banana
- 1/2 cup almond milk
- 1 tablespoon honey
- 1/2 teaspoon almond extract

Instructions:

1. Blend cherries, soaked almonds, banana, almond milk, honey, and almond extract until creamy.

2. Adjust sweetness and almond flavor to taste.

3. Enjoy the nutty goodness complemented by the sweetness of cherries!

Cooking Time: 5 minutes

18. Papaya Lime Zest

Ingredients:

- 1/2 cup papaya chunks
- 1/2 banana
- 1/2 lime (juiced)
- 1/2 cup coconut water
- 1/2 cup water
- Ice cubes

Instructions:

1. Blend papaya chunks, banana, lime juice, coconut water, and water until smooth.

2. Add ice cubes and blend for a cool and invigorating treat.

3. Savor the tropical flavors and zesty tang of papaya and lime!

Cooking Time: 5 minutes

19. Blueberry Walnut Bliss

Ingredients:

- 1/2 cup blueberries
- 1/4 cup walnuts
- 1/2 banana
- 1 cup almond milk
- 1 tablespoon chia seeds
- 1 teaspoon honey

Instructions:

1. Blend blueberries, walnuts, banana, almond milk, chia seeds, and honey until creamy.

2. Adjust sweetness and texture to your liking.

3. Delight in the rich flavors of blueberries and walnuts!

Cooking Time: 5 minutes

20. Orange Ginger Energizer

Ingredients:

- 1 orange (peeled and segmented)
- 1/2 inch ginger (peeled and grated)
- 1/2 banana
- 1/2 cup coconut water
- 1/2 cup water
- Ice cubes

Instructions:

1. Blend orange segments, grated ginger, banana, coconut water, and water until well combined.

2. Add ice cubes and blend for an energizing chill.

3. Get revitalized with the zing of orange and ginger!

Cooking Time: 5 minutes

21. Raspberry Avocado Dream

Ingredients:

- 1/2 cup raspberries
- 1/2 avocado
- 1/2 banana
- 1/2 cup almond milk
- 1 tablespoon chia seeds
- 1 teaspoon honey

Instructions:

1. Blend raspberries, avocado, banana, almond milk, chia seeds, and honey until creamy.

2. Adjust sweetness to taste with honey.

3. Revel in the creamy raspberry-avocado fusion!

Cooking Time: 5 minutes

22. Coconut Mango Basil

Ingredients:

- 1 cup mango chunks
- 1/4 cup fresh basil leaves
- 1/2 cup coconut milk
- 1/2 cup water
- Ice cubes

Instructions:

1. Blend mango chunks, basil leaves, coconut milk, and water until smooth.

2. Add ice cubes and blend for a cooling touch.

3. Enjoy the tropical embrace of coconut and mango with a hint of basil!

Cooking Time: 5 minutes

23. Pineapple Ginger Refresher

Ingredients:

-    1/2 cup pineapple chunks
-    1/2 inch ginger (peeled and grated)
-    1/2 banana
-    1/2 cup coconut water
-    1/2 cup water
-    Ice cubes

Instructions:

1. Blend pineapple chunks, grated ginger, banana, coconut water, and water until well mixed.

2. Add ice cubes and blend for a refreshing chill.

3. Recharge with the lively fusion of pineapple and ginger!

Cooking Time: 5 minutes

24. Mixed Berry Basil Bliss

Ingredients:

- 1/2 cup mixed berries (strawberries, blueberries, raspberries)
- 1/4 cup fresh basil leaves
- 1/2 banana
- 1/2 cup almond milk
- 1 tablespoon honey

Instructions:

1. Blend mixed berries, basil leaves, banana, almond milk, and honey until smooth.

2. Adjust sweetness with honey to your liking.

3. Experience the delightful balance of mixed berries and basil!

Cooking Time: 5 minutes

25. Almond Butter Banana Crunch

Ingredients:

- 1 banana
- 2 tablespoons almond butter
- 1/4 cup granola
- 1 cup almond milk
- 1 tablespoon honey
- Ice cubes

Instructions:

1. Blend banana, almond butter, granola, almond milk, and honey until creamy.

2. Add ice cubes and blend for a satisfying crunch.

3. Savor the nutty goodness of almond butter and the crunch of granola!

Cooking Time: 5 minutes

26. Spinach Kiwi Greenery

Ingredients:

- 2 kiwis (peeled and sliced)
- 1/2 banana
- 1 cup spinach
- 1/2 lime (juiced)
- 1/2 cup coconut water
- 1/2 cup water
- Ice cubes

Instructions:

1. Blend kiwis, banana, spinach, lime juice, coconut water, and water until smooth.

2. Add ice cubes and blend for a cooling effect.

3. Infuse your day with the vibrant green goodness of spinach and kiwi!

Cooking Time: 5 minutes

27. Chocolate Cherry Almond

Ingredients:

- 1/2 cup cherries (pitted)
- 1 tablespoon cocoa powder
- 1/4 cup almonds (soaked overnight)
- 1/2 banana
- 1 cup almond milk

Instructions:

1. Blend cherries, cocoa powder, soaked almonds, banana, and almond milk until smooth.

2. Adjust consistency to your preference.

3. Delight in the harmonious combination of chocolate, cherry, and almond!

Cooking Time: 5 minutes

28. Turmeric Mango Sunshine

Ingredients:

- 1 cup mango chunks
- 1/2 teaspoon turmeric powder
- 1/2 banana
- 1/2 orange (juiced)
- 1/2 cup coconut water
- Ice cubes

Instructions:

1. Blend mango chunks, turmeric powder, banana, orange juice, coconut water, and ice cubes until smooth.

2. Adjust turmeric and sweetness to taste.

3. Experience the sunny blend of mango and turmeric!

Cooking Time: 5 minutes

29. Blueberry Coconut Cream

Ingredients:

- 1/2 cup blueberries
- 1/2 banana
- 1/4 cup coconut cream
- 1 cup almond milk
- 1 tablespoon chia seeds
- 1 teaspoon honey

Instructions:

1. Blend blueberries, banana, coconut cream, almond milk, chia seeds, and honey until creamy.

2. Adjust creaminess and sweetness to your liking.

3. Enjoy the rich blueberry-coconut combination with a hint of creaminess!

Cooking Time: 5 minutes

30. Mango Mint Splash

Ingredients:

- 1 cup mango chunks
- 1/4 cup fresh mint leaves
- 1/2 banana
- 1/2 lime (juiced)
- 1/2 cup coconut water
- 1/2 cup water
- Ice cubes

Instructions:

1. Blend mango chunks, mint leaves, banana, lime juice, coconut water, and water until smooth.

2. Add ice cubes and blend for a cool and revitalizing splash.

3. Immerse yourself in the refreshing blend of mango and mint!

Cooking Time: 5 minutes

CONCLUSION

In the quest for optimal health and vitality, harnessing the power of nature's bounty can be an enlightening journey. The world of smoothies opens a gateway to nourishment, energy, and healing, especially when directed towards supporting thyroid health.

The intricate relationship between the thyroid gland and overall well-being underscores the importance of adopting a holistic approach to wellness.

Smoothies, infused with a carefully curated blend of fruits, vegetables, superfoods, and nutrients, have the potential to become a cornerstone of your thyroid-healing journey. Throughout this exploration, we've witnessed the myriad benefits that these flavorful concoctions offer to those seeking to rejuvenate their thyroid function.

The thyroid gland, a small but mighty regulator of metabolism and energy, thrives on specific nutrients such as iodine, selenium, zinc, and antioxidants. Incorporating these elements into your diet through smoothies provides a convenient and effective means to boost thyroid health.

Whether it's the thyroid-supportive qualities of iodine-rich sea vegetables, the antioxidant-rich properties of berries, or the hormone-balancing effects of adaptogens, each ingredient plays a crucial role in nurturing your thyroid.

Beyond the individual ingredients, the act of blending unlocks cellular barriers, making the nutrients more accessible and digestible.

This gentle processing allows your body to effortlessly absorb the goodness contained within the smoothie, ensuring that your thyroid receives the support it deserves.

The 30-day smoothie plan presented here is a versatile roadmap to explore a diverse array of flavors, textures, and combinations. From the vibrant greens of spinach and kale to the sweetness of tropical fruits like mango and pineapple, every sip holds the promise of nourishment.

Not only do these smoothies provide thyroid-specific nutrients, but they also cater to your taste preferences, making the journey enjoyable and sustainable.

However, it's important to remember that while smoothies can be a valuable tool in your thyroid-healing arsenal, they are most effective when integrated within a balanced and comprehensive approach to wellness. A holistic lifestyle includes factors like stress management, regular physical activity, adequate sleep, and personalized medical guidance.

Before embarking on any significant dietary changes, especially if you have an existing thyroid condition, it's wise to consult with a healthcare professional or registered dietitian. They can provide insights tailored to your individual health needs and ensure that the smoothie plan aligns with your overall wellness goals.

In conclusion, the marriage of nutrition and healing has never been as accessible and enjoyable as through the world of thyroid-healing smoothies. These vibrant elixirs have the potential to uplift not only your thyroid health but your entire well-being. As you sip on the carefully crafted blends, remember that you're nurturing a deeper connection with your body, embarking on a journey towards revitalization, and embracing the beauty of natural healing one delicious sip at a time.

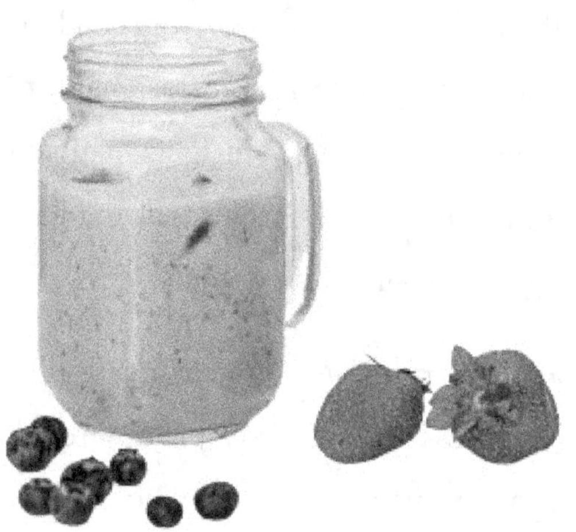